Amina Mnejja
Dhekra Toumi
Raja Faleh

Niemann Pick disease and pregnancy

Amina Mnejja
Dhekra Toumi
Raja Faleh

Niemann Pick disease and pregnancy

Imprint

Any brand names and product names mentioned in this book are subject to trademark, brand or patent protection and are trademarks or registered trademarks of their respective holders. The use of brand names, product names, common names, trade names, product descriptions etc. even without a particular marking in this work is in no way to be construed to mean that such names may be regarded as unrestricted in respect of trademark and brand protection legislation and could thus be used by anyone.

Cover image: www.ingimage.com

This book is a translation from the original published under ISBN 978-620-6-70974-9.

Publisher:
Sciencia Scripts
is a trademark of
Dodo Books Indian Ocean Ltd. and OmniScriptum S.R.L publishing group

120 High Road, East Finchley, London, N2 9ED, United Kingdom
Str. Armeneasca 28/1, office 1, Chisinau MD-2012, Republic of Moldova, Europe
Printed at: see last page
ISBN: 978-620-7-84884-3

Niemann Pick disease and pregnancy

Amina Mnejja

Dhekra Toumi

Raja Faleh

Service de Gynécologie Obstétrique Centre de
Maternité et de Néonatologie de Monastir

Biography

Amina Mnejja, obstetrics gynecology resident
Passionate about the Internet, reading and scientific research, she is fully committed to her specialty while cultivating her varied interests.

Key words

Niemann Pick, Deficiency, Sphyngomyelin, Sphingomyelinase acid, Enzymotherapy

Summary

Introduction

Acid sphingomyelinase (ASM) (sphingomyelin phosphodiesterase; EC 3.1.4.12) deficiency is an inborn error of metabolism that leads to the accumulation of sphingomyelin in cells and tissues, resulting in the clinical condition known as Niemann-Pick disease.

Key words

Niemann Pick, Deficiency, Sphyngomyelin, Sphingomyelinase acid, Enzymotherapy.

Case report

We report the case of an AB patient followed for Niemann Pick disease since childhood. She had an emergency caesarean section at 38 weeks for a post-traumatic retroplacental haematoma. uterine atony controlled by medical treatment. Simple postoperative course.

Conclusion

Since the discovery of the first patients with Niemann Pick disease over a century ago, enormous progress has been made in deciphering the pathophysiology of this disease and in developing new treatments.

Introduction

Acid sphingomyelinase (ASM) (sphingomyelin phosphodiesterase; EC 3.1.4.12) deficiency is an inborn error of metabolism that leads to the accumulation of sphingomyelin in cells and tissues, resulting in the clinical condition known as Niemann-Pick disease.

It is rare, with an estimated incidence of between 0.4 in 100,000 and 0.6 in 100,000 newborns (1,2,3).

Type A disease, which has a predilection for Ashkenazi Jews, is a severe neurodegenerative disease of childhood characterized by progressive psychomotor retardation, growth retardation, hepatosplenomegaly, cherry-red macula and death at the age of three or four.

Type B disease is pan-ethnic and characterized by hepatosplenomegaly, thrombocytopenia, interstitial lung disease and dyslipidemia, with most patients showing little or no neurological involvement. Liver dysfunction, retinal stigmata and growth retardation may also be present, but are more variable.

Type C disease is a genetically distinct condition resulting from a defect in intracellular cholesterol trafficking with secondary accumulation of glycosphingolipids.

No specific treatment has yet been established for Niemann Pick type A disease.

Conservative management protocols such as serum cholesterol reduction, oxygen supplementation and blood product transfusion can be implemented for Niemann Pick type B disease (4).

In addition, bone marrow transplantation has led to a reduction in spleen and liver volume and an increase in the number of peripheral blood cells, as well as a reduction in lung infiltration in some patients with Niemann Pick type B disease (5- 8).

Although enzyme replacement therapy is not part of the standard care protocol in Niemann Pick disease at present, researchers are working on early-phase clinical trials to evaluate the efficacy of enzyme replacement therapy in the early phase to evaluate the efficacy of recombinant ASM in the treatment of non-neurological manifestations in adults with Niemann Pick type B disease (7).

Post-partum hemorrhage (PPH) is the leading cause of maternal mortality worldwide.

Severe PPH can result in maternal mortality and morbidity, and is an obstetric emergency that must be meticulously managed (8).

Case report

Patient AB, 22 years old, primiparous, followed since childhood for Niemann-Pick disease.

She sought emergency care for pelvic pain and post-traumatic metrorrhagia following a fall down the stairs with an abdominal point of impact at 38 weeks' term.

Examination: uterine contracture, i.e. a real wooden belly and minimal black metrorrhagia.Ultrasound: positive cardiac activity.

Diagnosis of retroplacental hematoma with a live baby.

An emergency Caesarean section, complicated by uterine atony that was controlled by medical treatment (maximum dose of oxytocin, tranexamic acid and nalador).

A transfusion of labile blood products was performed.

Simple post-operative follow-up.

The baby has adapted well to life outside the womb.

Discussion

German pediatrician Albert Niemann described the first patient with Niemann Pick disease in 1914 in an Ashkenazi Jewish infant who presented with massive hepatosplenomegaly and a rapidly progressive neurodegenerative course that led to his death at the age of 18 months (9).

Type B patients show no obvious signs of CNS involvement, but hepatosplenomegaly may be profound and accompanied by signs of liver failure (10-12).

Serum triglycerides and LDL cholesterol are often elevated, while HDL cholesterol is low. The lungs are frequently affected in Niemann Pick type B disease, and pulmonary function is often compromised.

A reddish-brown halo may also surround the macula in the eyes of these patients, and in some cases a distinct cherry-red spot can be identified. Patients with intermediate findings between types A and B of this disease have also been described (13).

Niemann-Pick disease type C (NPC) is an autosomal recessive inherited lysosomal storage disease.

Completely distinct from types A and B (sphingomyelinase deficiency), it is mainly characterized by abnormalities in the intracellular transport of exogenous cholesterol, with lysosomal accumulation of unesterified cholesterol.

These abnormalities, present in cultured skin fibroblasts, enable biological diagnosis.

Joint genetic complementation and linkage studies have demonstrated that mutations in two distinct genes, NPC1 and NPC2, can cause NPC disease.

The NPC1 gene, located at 18q11 and identified in 1997, is mutated in over 95% of families. More recently, in 2000, HE1, located at 14q24.3, was recognized as the gene involved in the very rare second complementation group, and renamed NPC2.

The clinical and biochemical phenotypes of patients belonging to groups C1 or C2 are indistinguishable.

Niemann-Pick disease type C (NPC) is a rare lysosomal lipid storage disorder that manifests itself with a heterogeneous spectrum of clinical phenotypes, ranging from visceral to neurological to psychiatric symptoms.

Some of the common clinical manifestations of this neurovisceral disorder include hepatosplenomegaly, dystonia, ataxia, seizures and cognitive decline. Although the first symptoms can appear at any age, from the neonatal period to the sixth decade of life, the most common manifestation occurs in childhood, often leading to premature death. The etiology of this monogenetic disorder is attributed in around 95% of cases to autosomal recessive mutations in the NPC1 gene, while the remaining 5% of NPC patients carry mutations in the NPC2 gene. NPC1 encodes a large late endosome/lysosome protein with 13 transmembrane domains that interacts with the small soluble protein encoded by NPC2. The hydrophobic transfer model postulates that NPC2 transfers cholesterol to the N-terminal domain of NPC1. Their cooperative action ensures that cholesterol and other lipids are exported from late endosomes/lysosomes, thereby regulating cellular lipid homeostasis. The crystal structure of a large fragment of human NPC1 suggests that the "sterol-sensing domain" shapes a bidirectional cavity open to both the endosomal lumen and the light sheet of the lipid bilayer. Given these findings, cellular studies have shown that mutations in the sterol-sensing domain of NPC1 are associated with the accumulation of unesterified cholesterol. In addition to its proposed function as a lipid transporter, NPC1 regulates contact sites, facilitating lipid exchange between organelles.

Clinically, NPC disease is heterogeneous. In typical forms, the severity of the disease follows progressive neurological damage.

Neonatal manifestations, characterized by hepatosplenomegaly and cholestatic jaundice, are nevertheless present in almost 40% of patients. A rare neonatal form is characterized by lethal interstitial respiratory disease.

As insufficient SAM activity is characteristic of patients with type A and B, quantification of this enzyme activity in appropriate cells such as circulating leukocytes or cultured skin fibroblasts is the standard confirmatory diagnostic procedure (14,15).

SMPD1 gene sequencing can also be used to confirm the diagnosis, but should not be used as a first-line diagnostic indicator.

The presence of vacuolated cells in peripheral blood or bone marrow smears is also an indication of the disease, but is not diagnostic in the absence of enzymatic and/or genetic confirmation.

Enzyme tests on dried blood spots have also recently been developed to detect patients with NPD types A and B (15).

The differential diagnosis of type A and B patients must include Gaucher disease and type C Niemann Pick disease.

Biochemical and/or genetic tests carried out in a reliable laboratory can easily distinguish between these conditions.

Niemann Pick disease types A and B are inherited as recessive traits, and the degree of clinical involvement largely depends on the type of SMPD1 mutations inherited.

However, as the SMPD1 gene is subject to imprinting, phenotypes may also be due, at least in part, to the inheritance of specific mutations on maternal or paternal alleles.

Interestingly, abnormal clinical and laboratory findings have been reported in heterozygous individuals carrying a single mutation in the SMPD1 gene (16).

This could also be due to the inheritance of a single "severe" SMPD1 mutation on the maternal chromosome preferentially expressed.

Despite improvements in antenatal and postnatal care programs, PPH remains one of the leading causes of maternal mortality and morbidity in our country and worldwide (9).

PPH can result from a variety of obstetrical causes: uterine atony, maternal bleeding disorders, abnormal placentation, retained placenta, uterine inversion, etc. (10).

Niemann Pick type A and B are rare hereditary disorders of lysosomal storage (1, 2).

Patients with type B of this disease can survive into adulthood, and may present with various complications depending on the severity of the disease.

The main causes of death in patients with type B of this disease are heart failure and stroke, complications, bone marrow transplant complications, neurodegeneration and severe liver disease (1, 3).

Early onset of the disease and splenectomy are two main factors that increase the mortality rate, as both give an indication of the severity of the disease, according to recent studies of the disease (1, 3).

Trauma-related bleeding, postoperative hemorrhage, splenic vein tear and gastrointestinal hemorrhage/variceal bleeding were the leading causes of mortality.

Splenomegaly, However, to our knowledge, no case has been reported in the literature of a patient who died as a result of PPH.

Advances in the treatment of inborn errors of metabolism include recent clinical trials of enzyme replacement, substrate deprivation, pharmacological chaperone therapy and stem cell transplantation.

Conclusion

Since the discovery of the first patients with Niemann Pick disease over a century ago, enormous progress has been made in deciphering the pathophysiology of this disease and in developing new treatments.

Thanks to the contributions of Dr Brady and his colleagues, we now know that these patients have two distinct metabolic abnormalities: ASM deficiency in types A and B of this disease, and cholesterol esterification in type C. In this latter group, we also know that cholesterol esterification is a health risk factor.

In this latter group, we also know that there are two distinct gene and protein abnormalities that may be responsible for abnormal cholesterol metabolism (NPC1 and NPC2).

Leukopenia and thrombocytopenia tended to worsen over time, and the atherogenic lipid profile tended to remain markedly abnormal despite some normalization of triglyceride levels.

In addition, pulmonary function progressively deteriorated and serum transaminases remained elevated.

Unfortunately, many features of this progressive disease cannot be treated by available therapies.

Underlying metabolic abnormalities, such as enzyme replacement or gene therapy, may prove effective in treating the hematological, lipid, pulmonary and hepatic abnormalities of this disease.

References

1. Meikle P, Hopwood JJ, Clague AR, Carey WF. Prevalence of lysosomal storage disorders. JAMA1999;281:249–254. [PubMed: 9918480]

2. Poorthuis BJHM, Wevers RA, Kleijer WJ, et al. The frequency of lysosomal storage diseases in The Netherlands. Hum Genet 1999;105:151-156. [PubMed: 10480370]

3. Pinto R, Caseiro C, Lemos M, et al. Prevalence of lysosomal storage diseases in Portugal. Eur J Hum Genet 2004;12(2):87-92. [PubMed: 14685153]

4. M. M. McGovern,N. Lippa, E. Bagiella, E. H. Schuchman, R. J.Desnick, and M. P. Wasserstein, "Morbidity and mortality in type B Niemann-Pick disease," Genetics inMedicine, vol. 15, no. 8, pp. 618-623, 2013.

5. S. D. K. Kingma,O. A. Bodamer, and F. A. Wijburg, "Epidemiology and diagnosis of lysosomal storage disorders; Challenges of screening," Best Practice & Research Clinical Endocrinology & Metabolism, vol. 29, no. 2, pp. 145-157, 2015.

6. M. P. Wasserstein, A. Aron, S. E. Brodie, C. Simonaro, R. J.Desnick, and M. M. McGovern, "Acid sphingomyelinase deficiency: Prevalence and characterization of an intermediate phenotype of Niemann-Pick disease," Journal of Pediatrics, vol. 149, no. 4, pp. 554-559, 2006.

7.M. M. McGovern, M. P. Wasserstein, B. Kirmse et al, "Novel first-dose adverse drug reactions during a phase I trial of olipudase alfa (recombinant human acid sphingomyelinase) in adults with Niemann-Pick disease type B (acid sphingomyelinase deficiency)," Genetics in Medicine, vol. 18, no. 1, pp. 34-40, 2016.

8.L. Say, D. Chou, A. Gemmill et al, "Global causes of maternal death: a WHO systematic analysis," The Lancet Global Health, vol. 2, no. 6, pp. e323-e333, 2014.

9. Wasserstein MP, Desnick RJ, Schuchman EH, Hossain S. The natural history of type B Niemann-Pick disease: results from a 10-year longitudinal study. Pediatrics. 2004; 114:e672-e677. [PubMed: 15545621]

10. McGovern MM, Wasserstein MP, Giugliani R, Bembi B. A prospective cross-sectional survey study of the natural history of Niemann-Pick disease type B. Pediatrics. 2008; 122:e341-e349. [PubMed: 18625664]

11. Hollak CE, de Sonnaville ES, Cassiman D, Linthorst GE, Groener JE, Morava E, Wevers RA, Mannens M, Aerts JM, Meersseman W, Akkerman E, Niezen-Koning KE, Mulder MF, Visser G, Wiljburg FA, Lefeber D, Poorthuis BJ. Acid sphingomyelinase (ASM) deficiency patients in the Netherlands and Belgium: disease spectrum and natural course in

attenuated patients. Mol. Genet. Metab. 2012; 107:526-533. [PubMed: 22818240]

12. Pavlů-Pereira H, Asfaw B, Poupctová H, Ledvinová J, Sikora J, Vanier MT, Sandhoff K, Zeman J, Novotná Z, Chudoba D, Elleder M. Acid sphingomyelinase deficiency. Phenotype variability with prevalence of intermediate phenotype in a series of twenty-five Czech and Slovak patients. A multi-approach study. J. Inherit. Metab. Dis. 2005; 28:203-207. [PubMed: 15877209]

13. Gal AE, Brady RO, Hibbert SR. A practical chromogenic procedure for the detection of homozygotes and heterozygous carriers of Niemann-Pick disease. N. Engl. J. Med. 1975; 293:632-636. [PubMed: 239343]

14. He X, Chen F, Dagan A, Gatt S. A fluorescence-based, high-performance liquid chromatographic assay to determine acid sphingomyelinase activity and diagnose types A and B Niemann-Pick disease. Anal. Biochem. 2003; 314:116-120 [PubMed: 12633609]

15. Legnini E, Orsini JJ, Mühl A, Johnson B, Dajnoki A, Bodamer OA. Analysis of acid sphingomyelinase activity in dried blood spots using tandem mass spectrometry. Ann. Lab. Med. 2012; 32(5):319-323. [PubMed: 22950066

16. Lee CY, Krimbou L, Vincent J. Compound heterozygosity at the sphingomyelin phosphodiesterase-1 (SMPD1) gene is associated with low HDL cholesterol. Hum. Genet. 2003; 112:552-562. [PubMed: 12607113]

CONTENTS

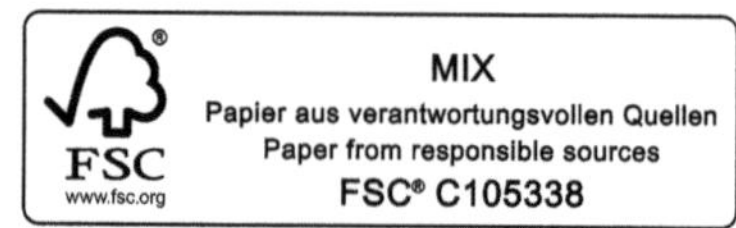

Printed by Books on Demand GmbH, Norderstedt / Germany